Free Book Offer:

Get How to be a Super Mom For Free

A Short Read is a type of book that is designed to be read in one quick sitting.

These no fluff books are perfect for people who want an overview about a subject in a short period of time.

Table of Contents

Natural Remedies for Enhancing Fertility

Natural Remedies for Enhancing Fertility

Are you looking for holistic methods to improve your fertility and increase your chances of conception? Look no further! In this article, we will explore various natural remedies that can help enhance fertility and promote reproductive health. From acupuncture to herbal supplements, exercise to diet, stress reduction techniques to alternative therapies, we will cover it all!

Acupuncture is an ancient practice that has been used for centuries to regulate hormones and improve reproductive health. By stimulating specific points on the body, acupuncture can help balance hormones, increase blood flow to the reproductive organs, and reduce stress. It is a safe and effective treatment option for both men and women who are trying to conceive.

Herbal supplements are another powerful tool in boosting fertility and balancing hormones. One such herb is Vitex, also known as Chaste Berry. This herb has been used for centuries to regulate menstrual cycles and promote ovulation. It can be taken in the form of capsules or tinctures, and it is best to consult with a healthcare professional for the appropriate dosage.

Another herbal supplement that can enhance fertility is Maca, a superfood known for its hormone-balancing properties. Maca can help regulate menstrual cycles, increase libido, and improve overall reproductive health. It can be consumed in powder or capsule form, and it is important to choose a high-quality organic product for maximum benefits.

Exercise and yoga are also crucial factors in improving fertility. Regular physical activity can help reduce stress, maintain a healthy weight, and improve overall reproductive function. Fertility yoga, in particular, focuses on specific poses that stimulate the reproductive organs and promote fertility. Incorporating cardiovascular exercise into your routine can also have a positive impact on fertility by improving blood flow and hormone balance.

A balanced diet and proper nutrition play a key role in enhancing fertility. Certain foods and nutrients have been found to boost fertility and improve reproductive health. Including foods rich in antioxidants, such as berries, leafy greens, and nuts, can protect the eggs and sperm from oxidative damage. On the other hand, it is important to limit the consumption of sugar and processed foods, as they can negatively affect fertility.

Stress reduction techniques, such as meditation and aromatherapy, can also have a profound impact on fertility. Meditation helps calm the mind, reduce stress, and balance hormones, creating a more fertile environment for conception. Aromatherapy, using essential oils such as lavender or chamomile, can promote relaxation and improve reproductive health.

Exploring alternative therapies can also be beneficial for enhancing fertility. Mayan abdominal massage is an ancient technique that improves blood flow to the reproductive organs, helping to balance hormones and promote fertility. Castor oil packs are another natural remedy that can detoxify the body and improve fertility by reducing inflammation and increasing circulation to the reproductive organs.

Environmental factors can also have a significant impact on fertility. Endocrine disruptors, which are chemicals found in everyday products, can disrupt hormonal balance and interfere with reproductive function. It is important to minimize exposure to these toxins by choosing natural and organic products and creating a fertility-friendly home environment.

When it comes to male fertility, antioxidant supplements can play a crucial role in improving sperm quality and fertility. Antioxidants protect the sperm from oxidative damage, which can affect its motility and viability. Additionally, adopting healthy lifestyle habits, including a balanced diet, regular exercise, and stress reduction techniques, can greatly enhance male fertility.

If natural remedies do not yield the desired results, it may be time to seek professional help. Natural fertility specialists, such as naturopathic doctors and holistic practitioners, can provide personalized treatment plans to address specific fertility issues. Assisted reproductive technologies, such as in vitro fertilization (IVF) or intrauterine insemination (IUI), are also options to consider, depending on individual circumstances.

Lastly, the importance of emotional support and connecting with others on a fertility journey should not be underestimated. Joining a fertility support group can provide both emotional and informational support, allowing individuals to share their experiences and learn from others. Online resources and forums are also valuable platforms for connecting with a wider community and finding support during the fertility journey.

In conclusion, there are numerous natural remedies available to enhance fertility and increase the chances of conception. By exploring holistic methods such as acupuncture, herbal supplements, exercise and yoga, diet and nutrition, stress reduction techniques, alternative therapies, environmental factors, and seeking professional help, individuals can take proactive steps towards improving their reproductive health and realizing their dreams of starting a family.

Acupuncture

Acupuncture is an ancient practice that has been used for centuries to promote overall health and well-being. It involves the insertion of thin needles into specific points on the body to stimulate the flow of energy, known as Qi. In the context of fertility, acupuncture can be a powerful tool for regulating hormones and improving reproductive health.

One of the key ways acupuncture can enhance fertility is by balancing hormones. Hormonal imbalances can disrupt the menstrual cycle and interfere with ovulation, making it more difficult to conceive. Acupuncture works by stimulating the release of hormones that regulate the menstrual cycle, such as follicle-stimulating hormone (FSH) and luteinizing hormone (LH). By promoting hormonal balance, acupuncture can help regulate the menstrual cycle and improve the chances of ovulation.

In addition to hormone regulation, acupuncture can also improve blood flow to the reproductive organs. This is important because adequate blood flow is essential for optimal reproductive function. When blood flow is compromised, it can lead to issues such as poor egg quality and uterine lining thickness. Acupuncture helps to increase blood flow to the uterus and ovaries, improving their overall health and function.

Moreover, acupuncture can reduce stress, which is a common factor that can negatively impact fertility. Stress can disrupt hormonal balance and interfere with the reproductive process. Acupuncture has been shown to stimulate the release of endorphins, which are natural painkillers and mood boosters. By promoting relaxation and reducing stress, acupuncture can create a more favorable environment for conception.

It is important to note that acupuncture is not a standalone treatment for infertility. It is often used in conjunction with other holistic approaches, such as herbal supplements and lifestyle modifications. Additionally, it is recommended to seek the guidance of a qualified acupuncturist who specializes in fertility to ensure the best results.

Herbal Supplements

Herbal supplements have long been used as natural remedies for enhancing fertility and balancing hormones. These powerful plants contain compounds that can support reproductive health and increase the chances of conception. By incorporating herbal supplements into your daily routine, you can harness the benefits of nature to optimize your fertility journey.

One popular herb for boosting fertility is Vitex, also known as Chaste Tree Berry. This herb has been used for centuries to regulate menstrual cycles and promote ovulation. Vitex works by stimulating the release of luteinizing hormone (LH), which is essential for the maturation of eggs and the production of progesterone. By balancing hormone levels, Vitex can help regulate the menstrual cycle and increase the chances of successful conception.

Another powerful herbal supplement is Maca, a superfood native to the Andes Mountains. Maca has been used for centuries to enhance fertility by balancing hormones and increasing libido. This adaptogenic herb can help regulate the endocrine system, which is responsible for hormone production and regulation. By supporting hormonal balance, Maca can improve fertility and increase the chances of conception.

When incorporating herbal supplements into your fertility regimen, it's important to consult with a healthcare professional or a qualified herbalist. They can guide you in choosing the right herbs and dosages for your specific needs. Additionally, it's important to note that herbal supplements may take time to show results, so patience and consistency are key. With the power of herbs on your side, you can boost your fertility naturally and increase your chances of achieving the dream of parenthood.

Vitex

Vitex, also known as Chaste Tree Berry, is a powerful herb that has been used for centuries to regulate menstrual cycles and promote ovulation. This natural remedy has gained popularity among women seeking to enhance their fertility and increase their chances of conception.

One of the key benefits of Vitex is its ability to balance hormones. It acts on the pituitary gland, which is responsible for regulating the release of hormones involved in the menstrual cycle. By stimulating the production of luteinizing hormone (LH) and inhibiting the release of follicle-stimulating hormone (FSH), Vitex helps to promote regular ovulation and regulate the menstrual cycle.

Additionally, Vitex has been found to have a positive impact on progesterone levels. Progesterone is a hormone that plays a crucial role in preparing the uterus for implantation and maintaining a healthy pregnancy. By increasing progesterone levels, Vitex can improve the chances of successful implantation and reduce the risk of miscarriage.

Furthermore, Vitex has been shown to have a calming effect on the nervous system, which can be beneficial for women experiencing symptoms of PMS or hormonal imbalances. It can help to alleviate mood swings, irritability, and breast tenderness, making the menstrual cycle more manageable.

It is important to note that Vitex is not a quick fix solution and may take several months to show its full effects. It is recommended to take Vitex consistently for at least three to six months to experience its maximum benefits. It is also advisable to consult with a healthcare professional before starting any herbal supplement, especially if you are taking any medications or have any underlying medical conditions.

In conclusion, Vitex is a natural remedy that can be used to regulate menstrual cycles and promote ovulation. Its hormone-balancing properties and ability to increase progesterone levels make it a valuable tool for women looking to enhance their fertility. However, it is important to approach the use of Vitex with patience and consult with a healthcare professional for personalized advice and guidance.

Maca

Maca, also known as Peruvian ginseng, is a powerful superfood that has been used for centuries to enhance fertility. This incredible root vegetable is packed with nutrients and bioactive compounds that can have a positive impact on reproductive health.

One of the key benefits of maca is its ability to balance hormones. Hormonal imbalances can often be a contributing factor to infertility, and maca works by stimulating the endocrine system and regulating hormone production. This can be particularly beneficial for women with irregular menstrual cycles or hormonal disorders such as polycystic ovary syndrome (PCOS).

In addition to balancing hormones, maca has also been shown to increase libido. This can be especially helpful for couples who are trying to conceive, as a healthy sex drive is important for successful conception. Maca works by increasing blood flow to the pelvic region and improving sexual function.

Furthermore, maca is rich in essential nutrients such as vitamins, minerals, and antioxidants. These nutrients play a crucial role in reproductive health and can support the development of healthy eggs and sperm. Maca is particularly high in iron, which is important for maintaining optimal fertility.

There are several ways to incorporate maca into your diet. It is available in powder form, which can be added to smoothies, yogurt, or baked goods. You can also find maca capsules or tablets for easy consumption. It is recommended to start with a small dosage and gradually increase it to find the right amount for your body.

It's important to note that while maca has been shown to have positive effects on fertility, it is not a miracle cure. It should be used in conjunction with a healthy lifestyle, including a balanced diet, regular exercise, and stress management. If you have any underlying health conditions or concerns, it's always best to consult with a healthcare professional before incorporating maca into your routine.

Exercise and Yoga

Exercise and yoga play a crucial role in enhancing fertility by promoting physical activity and reducing stress levels. Engaging in regular physical activity not only improves overall health but also increases the chances of conception. When we exercise, our body releases endorphins, which are known as "feel-good" hormones. These endorphins help to reduce stress and anxiety, which can have a negative impact on fertility.

One way to incorporate exercise into your routine is through fertility yoga. Fertility yoga involves specific poses and movements that target the reproductive organs and stimulate blood flow to the pelvic area. This increased blood flow can improve the health of the reproductive system and enhance fertility. Some fertility yoga poses include the butterfly pose, the reclining bound angle pose, and the supported bridge pose.

In addition to fertility yoga, cardiovascular exercise is also beneficial for fertility. Regular aerobic exercise, such as jogging, swimming, or cycling, improves blood circulation and increases oxygen flow throughout the body. This can enhance the health of the reproductive organs and promote a regular menstrual cycle.

It is important to note that while exercise is beneficial for fertility, it is essential to strike a balance. Excessive exercise or intense workouts can actually have a negative impact on fertility. It is recommended to engage in moderate exercise for about 30 minutes a day, five days a week.

Incorporating exercise and yoga into your daily routine can not only improve your physical health but also enhance your fertility by reducing stress levels and promoting a healthy reproductive system. So, lace up those sneakers or roll out your yoga mat and get moving!

Fertility Yoga

Fertility Yoga is a powerful practice that can help stimulate reproductive organs and promote fertility. By incorporating specific yoga poses into your routine, you can enhance blood flow to the pelvic region, balance hormones, and create a nurturing environment for conception.

One of the key benefits of Fertility Yoga is its ability to reduce stress and promote relaxation. Stress can have a negative impact on fertility by disrupting hormonal balance and affecting ovulation. Fertility Yoga incorporates deep breathing techniques and gentle stretching to calm the mind and release tension in the body.

Some specific yoga poses that are known to support fertility include:

- **Baddha Konasana (Butterfly Pose)** - This pose helps open up the hips and stimulate the ovaries.
- **Supported Bridge Pose** - This pose improves blood circulation to the reproductive organs and helps balance hormones.

- **Legs Up the Wall Pose** - This pose allows for better blood flow to the pelvic region and can help reduce stress.
- **Reclining Bound Angle Pose** - This pose stretches the groin and stimulates the reproductive organs.

It's important to note that Fertility Yoga should be practiced in conjunction with other holistic approaches to enhance fertility. It is not a standalone solution, but rather a complementary practice that can support overall reproductive health.

By incorporating Fertility Yoga into your routine, you can create a positive mindset, reduce stress, and optimize your body for conception. Remember to always listen to your body and consult with a qualified yoga instructor before starting any new exercise program.

Cardiovascular Exercise

Regular aerobic exercise has numerous benefits for improving fertility. Engaging in cardiovascular exercises such as running, swimming, or cycling can positively impact reproductive health in both men and women. Let's explore the benefits of regular aerobic exercise in enhancing fertility.

1. Enhanced Blood Flow: Cardiovascular exercise increases blood circulation throughout the body, including the reproductive organs. This improved blood flow ensures that

the reproductive organs receive an adequate supply of oxygen and nutrients, promoting their optimal function.

2. Hormonal Balance: Regular aerobic exercise helps regulate hormone levels in the body. It can reduce excess levels of estrogen, which can interfere with ovulation in women. In men, exercise can increase testosterone levels, which is essential for sperm production.

3. Weight Management: Maintaining a healthy weight is crucial for fertility. Regular cardiovascular exercise helps in managing weight by burning calories and reducing excess body fat. Obesity and being underweight can both negatively impact fertility.

4. Stress Reduction: Exercise is known to be a great stress reliever. It stimulates the release of endorphins, which are natural mood boosters. By reducing stress levels, regular aerobic exercise can help balance hormones and improve fertility.

5. Improved Ovulation: For women with irregular menstrual cycles or ovulation issues, regular aerobic exercise can help regulate the menstrual cycle and promote regular ovulation. This, in turn, increases the chances of conception.

6. Increased Sperm Quality: Men who engage in regular cardiovascular exercise often have better sperm quality. Exercise helps in reducing oxidative stress, which can damage sperm DNA. Additionally, it improves sperm motility and count, increasing the chances of successful fertilization.

It is important to note that while regular aerobic exercise can be beneficial for fertility, excessive exercise or overtraining can have the opposite effect. It is essential to strike a balance and engage in moderate-intensity exercises for optimal results.

Incorporating cardiovascular exercise into your daily routine can have a positive impact on your fertility journey. However, it is always advisable to consult with a healthcare professional or fertility specialist before starting any new exercise regimen, especially if you have any underlying health conditions or concerns.

Diet and Nutrition

Diet and nutrition play a crucial role in enhancing fertility and increasing the chances of conception. A balanced diet that includes specific nutrients can support reproductive health and optimize hormonal balance. Here are some key factors to consider when it comes to diet and fertility:

- **Foods to Boost Fertility:** Certain foods are known to have fertility-enhancing properties. For example, foods rich in antioxidants, such as berries, leafy greens, and nuts, can help protect eggs and sperm from oxidative damage. Additionally, incorporating foods high in omega-3 fatty acids, such as salmon and chia seeds, can support hormone production and improve fertility.

- **The Impact of Sugar and Processed Foods:** Consuming excessive amounts of sugar and processed foods can negatively affect fertility. These foods can cause inflammation in the body and disrupt hormonal balance. It is important to limit the intake of sugary beverages, processed snacks, and refined carbohydrates, and instead focus on whole, nutrient-dense foods.

In addition to specific foods, it is essential to maintain a well-balanced diet that includes a variety of nutrients. Some key nutrients that support fertility include:

- **Folic Acid:** This B-vitamin is crucial for healthy egg and sperm development. It can be found in leafy greens, citrus fruits, and fortified grains.
- **Iron:** Iron is important for blood flow and reproductive health. Good sources of iron include lean meats, beans, and dark leafy greens.
- **Calcium:** Calcium is essential for reproductive hormone function. Dairy products, fortified plant-based milks, and leafy greens are excellent sources of calcium.
- **Zinc:** Zinc is involved in hormone production and sperm development. Foods rich in zinc include oysters, lean meats, and pumpkin seeds.

It is important to consult with a healthcare professional or a registered dietitian to create a personalized fertility-enhancing diet plan. They can provide guidance on the specific nutrient needs and recommend a well-rounded diet that supports reproductive health.

Foods to Boost Fertility

When it comes to enhancing fertility, the power of nutrition should not be underestimated. Certain foods are known to possess fertility-enhancing properties and can provide the necessary nutrients to support reproductive health. Including these foods in your diet can increase your chances of conception and promote overall fertility.

Here are some fertility-boosting foods and nutrients to incorporate into your daily meals:

- **Folate:** Found in leafy greens, citrus fruits, and legumes, folate is essential for healthy egg development and can reduce the risk of birth defects.
- **Omega-3 fatty acids:** Foods rich in omega-3 fatty acids, such as salmon, walnuts, and flaxseeds, can improve hormone production and regulate menstrual cycles.
- **Antioxidants:** Berries, dark chocolate, and green tea are packed with antioxidants that protect reproductive cells from damage caused by free radicals.

- **Iron:** Iron-rich foods like lean meats, spinach, and lentils can prevent anemia and promote optimal fertility.
- **Zinc:** Found in oysters, pumpkin seeds, and lean meats, zinc is crucial for hormone regulation and sperm production.
- **Vitamin D:** Foods fortified with vitamin D, such as milk and fortified cereals, can improve fertility by enhancing the production of sex hormones.

In addition to these specific nutrients, it's important to maintain a balanced diet that includes a variety of fruits, vegetables, whole grains, and lean proteins. Avoiding processed foods, excessive caffeine, and alcohol can also support fertility.

Remember, while incorporating these foods into your diet can be beneficial, it's always best to consult with a healthcare professional or a registered dietitian to ensure you're meeting your individual nutritional needs for fertility enhancement.

The Impact of Sugar and Processed Foods

Sugar and processed foods have become a staple in many people's diets, but their impact on fertility should not be underestimated. Consuming an unhealthy diet high in sugar and processed foods can have detrimental effects on reproductive health and decrease the chances of conception.

One of the main ways that sugar and processed foods can negatively affect fertility is by causing hormonal imbalances. These foods are often high in refined carbohydrates, which quickly raise blood sugar levels and lead to insulin spikes. This can disrupt the delicate balance of hormones in the body, including those involved in the menstrual cycle and ovulation.

Furthermore, a diet high in sugar and processed foods can lead to inflammation in the body. Chronic inflammation can interfere with the normal functioning of reproductive organs and impair fertility. Inflammation has been linked to conditions such as polycystic ovary syndrome (PCOS) and endometriosis, both of which can contribute to infertility.

Additionally, a diet that is lacking in essential nutrients due to the overconsumption of sugar and processed foods can also negatively impact fertility. These foods are often low in vitamins, minerals, and antioxidants that are crucial for reproductive health. Adequate intake of nutrients such as folate, zinc, and vitamin D is essential for healthy egg and sperm development, as well as proper hormone regulation.

It is important to note that not all sugars and processed foods are created equal. Highly processed foods often contain added sugars, artificial sweeteners, and unhealthy fats that can have a more significant impact on fertility. Opting for a diet rich in whole, unprocessed foods such as fruits, vegetables, lean proteins, and whole grains can help support reproductive health.

In conclusion, the impact of sugar and processed foods on fertility should not be overlooked. These dietary choices can disrupt hormonal balance, contribute to inflammation, and deprive the body of essential nutrients. Making healthier dietary choices by reducing sugar and processed food intake can play a significant role in enhancing fertility and increasing the chances of conception.

Stress Reduction Techniques

Stress can have a significant impact on fertility, as it can disrupt hormonal balance and interfere with the reproductive system. That's why it's crucial to explore stress reduction techniques that can help improve fertility. By incorporating relaxation methods into your daily routine, you can not only reduce stress but also enhance your chances of conceiving.

One effective stress reduction technique is meditation. This ancient practice has been shown to calm the mind and balance hormones, creating a more fertile environment within the body. Taking just a few minutes each day to sit in a quiet space and focus on your breath can work wonders for reducing stress levels and promoting fertility.

Aromatherapy is another powerful tool for stress reduction and fertility enhancement. Essential oils such as lavender, chamomile, and ylang-ylang have calming properties that can help relax the body and mind. You can use these oils in a diffuser, add a few drops to your bath, or even apply them topically for a soothing effect.

In addition to these techniques, it's important to prioritize self-care and engage in activities that bring you joy and relaxation. Whether it's taking a warm bath, practicing gentle yoga, or indulging in a hobby you love, finding ways to unwind and destress is essential for improving fertility.

Remember, reducing stress not only benefits your overall well-being but also increases your chances of conceiving. By incorporating stress reduction techniques into your daily routine, you can create a more fertile environment within your body and enhance your fertility naturally.

Meditation

Meditation is a powerful practice that can have a profound impact on fertility. By calming the mind and reducing stress, meditation helps to balance hormones and create an optimal environment for conception. When we are stressed, our bodies release cortisol, a hormone that can interfere with reproductive function. By incorporating meditation into your daily routine, you can lower cortisol levels and promote hormonal balance.

During meditation, you focus your attention and eliminate the stream of thoughts that often clutter the mind. This state of deep relaxation allows the body to activate its natural healing mechanisms and restore balance. Regular meditation practice can also improve blood flow to the reproductive organs, enhancing their function and increasing the chances of conception.

To get started with meditation, find a quiet and comfortable space where you can sit or lie down. Close your eyes and take deep, slow breaths. Focus on your breath as you inhale and exhale, letting go of any tension or stress with each breath. Allow your mind to become still and observe any thoughts or sensations that arise without judgment. With practice, meditation can become a valuable tool for reducing stress and enhancing fertility.

Aromatherapy

Aromatherapy is a holistic approach to reducing stress and promoting reproductive health through the use of essential oils. Essential oils are highly concentrated plant extracts that have been used for centuries for their therapeutic properties. When inhaled or applied topically, these oils can have a profound impact on our physical and emotional well-being.

Essential oils can be used in a variety of ways to support fertility. One popular method is through diffusing oils in a room or using them in a bath. This allows the scent to be inhaled, which can have a calming effect on the mind and body. Some oils that are particularly beneficial for reducing stress and promoting relaxation include lavender, chamomile, and ylang-ylang.

In addition to inhalation, essential oils can also be applied topically through massage or diluted in carrier oils. This allows the oils to be absorbed through the skin, where they can have a direct impact on the reproductive system. Certain oils, such as clary sage and geranium, are known for their hormone-balancing properties and can be used to support overall reproductive health.

It's important to note that essential oils should be used with caution and under the guidance of a trained aromatherapist or healthcare professional. Some oils may have contraindications or interactions with certain medications, so it's important to do your research and consult with a professional before incorporating aromatherapy into your fertility journey.

In summary, aromatherapy is a natural and effective way to reduce stress and promote reproductive health. By using essential oils in diffusers, baths, or through massage, individuals can experience the benefits of these powerful plant extracts. However, it's important to use caution and seek professional guidance to ensure safe and effective use of essential oils.

Alternative Therapies

Alternative therapies offer a unique approach to enhancing fertility naturally. While they may not be as widely known or practiced as conventional methods, these therapies can provide valuable support to individuals and couples on their fertility journey. Let's explore some of these lesser-known therapies and their potential benefits.

Mayan Abdominal Massage: This ancient technique focuses on gently massaging the abdomen to improve blood flow to the reproductive organs. By increasing circulation and reducing tension, Mayan abdominal massage can help promote a healthy menstrual cycle and support overall reproductive health.

Castor Oil Packs: Castor oil packs involve applying a cloth soaked in warm castor oil to the lower abdomen. This therapy is believed to help detoxify the body, reduce inflammation, and improve fertility. The castor oil penetrates deep into the tissues, stimulating circulation and supporting the body's natural detoxification processes.

These alternative therapies can be used in conjunction with other fertility-enhancing methods to create a holistic approach to reproductive health. It's important to consult with a qualified practitioner experienced in these therapies to ensure proper technique and guidance.

Mayan Abdominal Massage

Mayan Abdominal Massage is an ancient technique that has been used for centuries to improve blood flow to the reproductive organs. This holistic therapy originated from the Mayan civilization and is based on the belief that the abdomen is the center of our health and vitality. By gently manipulating the abdominal area, this massage technique aims to release tension, improve circulation, and restore balance to the reproductive system.

The Mayan Abdominal Massage focuses on specific techniques that target the uterus, ovaries, and fallopian tubes. The therapist uses gentle, rhythmic movements to stimulate blood flow and encourage the proper positioning of these organs. By doing so, this massage technique can help alleviate blockages, reduce inflammation, and promote a healthy environment for conception.

One of the key benefits of Mayan Abdominal Massage is its ability to improve blood circulation to the reproductive organs. This increased blood flow brings fresh oxygen and nutrients to the area, while also removing toxins and waste products. By enhancing circulation, this massage technique can help nourish the reproductive organs and promote their optimal function.

In addition to improving blood flow, Mayan Abdominal Massage can also help to relieve tension and reduce stress in the abdominal area. Stress and tension can negatively impact fertility by disrupting the hormonal balance and creating an unfavorable environment for conception. By releasing tension and promoting relaxation, this massage technique can help restore harmony to the reproductive system and enhance fertility.

Mayan Abdominal Massage is a non-invasive and natural approach to improving fertility. It can be beneficial for individuals who are trying to conceive naturally or undergoing assisted reproductive technologies. However, it is important to note that this technique should be performed by a trained and experienced therapist who specializes in Mayan Abdominal Massage.

If you are considering Mayan Abdominal Massage as part of your fertility journey, it is recommended to consult with a qualified practitioner who can assess your specific needs and provide personalized guidance. They can tailor the massage to address any underlying issues or imbalances in your reproductive system, increasing the effectiveness of the treatment.

Overall, Mayan Abdominal Massage offers a holistic and gentle approach to improving blood flow to the reproductive organs. By promoting circulation, reducing tension, and restoring balance, this ancient technique can enhance fertility and increase the chances of conception. If you are seeking a natural and non-invasive method to support your fertility journey, Mayan Abdominal Massage may be worth exploring.

Castor Oil Packs

Castor oil packs are a natural and effective method for detoxifying the body and improving fertility. These packs involve applying a cloth soaked in warm castor oil to the abdomen and covering it with a plastic wrap or towel. The pack is then left on for a specified period of time, usually ranging from 30 minutes to a few hours.

One of the main benefits of castor oil packs is their ability to stimulate blood circulation and lymphatic drainage in the reproductive organs. This increased circulation helps to remove toxins and promote the health of the uterus, ovaries, and fallopian tubes. By detoxifying the reproductive system, castor oil packs can improve the overall function and balance of the reproductive organs, increasing the chances of conception.

In addition to detoxification, castor oil packs also have anti-inflammatory properties. They can help reduce inflammation in the reproductive organs, which is often a contributing factor to fertility issues. By reducing inflammation, castor oil packs create a more optimal environment for conception and implantation of a fertilized egg.

Using castor oil packs regularly can also help to relieve pelvic congestion and reduce the risk of developing uterine fibroids or ovarian cysts. The gentle heat from the pack can help to relax the muscles and tissues in the pelvic area, promoting better circulation and reducing congestion.

To use a castor oil pack, start by applying a generous amount of castor oil to a clean cloth. Place the cloth on the lower abdomen and cover it with plastic wrap or a towel to trap the heat. You can use a heating pad or hot water bottle to further warm the pack and enhance its effects. Relax and allow the pack to work its magic for the recommended time. Afterward, remove the pack and cleanse the skin with a gentle soap and warm water.

It's important to note that castor oil packs should not be used during pregnancy or menstruation. If you have any underlying health conditions or concerns, it's always best to consult with a healthcare professional before incorporating castor oil packs into your fertility routine.

In conclusion, castor oil packs are a natural and accessible method for detoxifying the body and improving fertility. By promoting circulation, reducing inflammation, and relieving pelvic congestion, these packs can enhance the overall health of the reproductive system and increase the chances of conception. Consider adding castor oil packs to your fertility regimen to support your journey towards parenthood.

Environmental Factors

Environmental factors play a significant role in fertility and can have a profound impact on reproductive health. Exposure to environmental toxins can disrupt hormonal balance, impair sperm and egg quality, and decrease fertility. It is essential to understand these factors and take steps to minimize exposure to protect and enhance fertility.

Chemicals known as endocrine disruptors are found in everyday products such as plastics, pesticides, and personal care items. These chemicals can interfere with the normal functioning of hormones in the body, leading to fertility issues. To minimize exposure to endocrine disruptors, it is crucial to choose products that are free from harmful chemicals. Opt for organic and natural alternatives whenever possible and avoid using plastic containers for food and beverages.

Creating a fertility-friendly home environment is also crucial. This involves reducing exposure to toxins in the air, water, and household products. Use air purifiers to improve indoor air quality, filter drinking water to remove contaminants, and opt for natural cleaning products that are free from harsh chemicals. Additionally, avoid smoking and limit alcohol consumption, as these habits can also negatively impact fertility.

It is important to be aware of the potential environmental toxins in your surroundings and take proactive measures to minimize exposure. By making small changes to your lifestyle and environment, you can create a healthier and more fertility-friendly space that supports your reproductive health.

Endocrine Disruptors

Endocrine disruptors are chemicals found in everyday products that can have a detrimental effect on hormonal balance and fertility. These chemicals can interfere with the body's endocrine system, which is responsible for regulating hormones that play a crucial role in reproductive health.

Common sources of endocrine disruptors include household cleaning products, personal care items, plastics, and pesticides. These chemicals can mimic or block the actions of natural hormones in the body, leading to hormonal imbalances and potentially affecting fertility.

Research has shown that exposure to endocrine disruptors can have various negative effects on reproductive health. For women, these chemicals can disrupt menstrual cycles, interfere with ovulation, and affect the quality of eggs. In men, endocrine disruptors can impact sperm production, motility, and overall sperm quality.

It is important to be aware of the potential sources of endocrine disruptors and take steps to minimize exposure. Reading product labels and choosing items that are free from harmful chemicals can help reduce the risk. Opting for natural cleaning products, using glass or stainless steel containers instead of plastic, and choosing organic foods can also make a difference.

Additionally, it is crucial to create a fertility-friendly environment at home. This can involve avoiding the use of synthetic fragrances, which often contain endocrine-disrupting chemicals, and opting for natural alternatives. Using air purifiers and regularly ventilating the home can also help reduce exposure to indoor pollutants.

By understanding the impact of endocrine disruptors and taking proactive steps to minimize exposure, individuals can support their hormonal balance and enhance their fertility.

Creating a Fertility-Friendly Home

Creating a Fertility-Friendly Home

When it comes to enhancing fertility, it's important to consider the environment in which you live. Our homes can be filled with hidden toxins that can disrupt hormonal balance and negatively impact fertility. By taking steps to reduce exposure to these toxins, you can create a fertility-friendly home that supports your reproductive health. Here are some tips to get you started:

- Avoid using chemical-based cleaning products and opt for natural alternatives. Many conventional cleaning products contain harmful ingredients that can interfere with hormonal function. Look for eco-friendly options or make your own cleaners using simple ingredients like vinegar, baking soda, and essential oils.
- Choose organic and non-toxic household products. From furniture to bedding, many items in our homes can off-gas harmful chemicals that can affect fertility. Opt for organic and natural materials whenever possible, and avoid products that contain flame retardants, phthalates, and other harmful substances.
- Filter your tap water. Tap water can contain traces of chemicals and heavy metals that can disrupt hormonal balance. Invest in a high-quality water filter to remove these contaminants and ensure that you're drinking clean, pure water.
- Minimize exposure to electromagnetic radiation. Electronic devices emit electromagnetic fields (EMFs) that can potentially affect fertility. Keep your distance from devices like laptops and cell phones, especially when trying to conceive. Consider turning off Wi-Fi at night and creating a

technology-free bedroom for better sleep and reproductive health.
- Improve indoor air quality. Indoor air can be more polluted than outdoor air, so it's essential to improve air circulation and reduce exposure to toxins. Open windows regularly to let fresh air in, use air purifiers to filter out pollutants, and avoid smoking or allowing others to smoke in your home.

By implementing these tips, you can create a safe and healthy environment that supports your fertility journey. Remember, small changes can make a big difference when it comes to reducing exposure to toxins and improving reproductive health.

Male Fertility

When it comes to fertility, it's not just women who need to focus on their reproductive health. Men play a crucial role in conception, and their fertility can also be influenced by various factors. If you're looking to enhance male fertility and improve sperm quality, there are natural remedies that can help.

1. Antioxidant Supplements: Antioxidants are known for their ability to protect the body against oxidative damage caused by free radicals. When it comes to male fertility, antioxidants can play a significant role in improving sperm quality. Supplements such as vitamin C, vitamin E, and selenium have been shown to enhance sperm count, motility, and morphology.

2. Healthy Lifestyle Habits: Adopting a healthy lifestyle can have a positive impact on male fertility. It's essential to maintain a balanced diet rich in fruits, vegetables, whole grains, and lean proteins. Regular exercise can also improve sperm production and quality. Additionally, stress reduction techniques such as meditation and yoga can help balance hormones and promote better reproductive health.

3. Avoiding Environmental Toxins: Environmental toxins can have a detrimental effect on male fertility. Exposure to chemicals found in everyday products, such as pesticides, plastics, and certain cleaning agents, can disrupt hormonal balance and sperm production. Minimizing exposure to these toxins by using natural and organic products can help protect male fertility.

4. Adequate Sleep: Getting enough sleep is crucial for overall health, including male fertility. Lack of sleep can disrupt hormonal balance and affect sperm production. Aim for seven to eight hours of quality sleep each night to support optimal reproductive function.

5. Herbal Supplements: Certain herbal supplements have been traditionally used to enhance male fertility. Tribulus terrestris, maca root, and ashwagandha are known for their potential benefits in improving sperm count, motility, and quality. However, it's important to consult with a healthcare professional before starting any herbal supplements.

By incorporating these natural remedies into your lifestyle, you can support male fertility and improve sperm quality. Remember, it's always essential to consult with a healthcare professional for personalized advice and guidance on enhancing male fertility.

Antioxidant Supplements

Antioxidant supplements play a crucial role in protecting sperm from oxidative damage and improving fertility. Oxidative stress occurs when there is an imbalance between the production of free radicals and the body's ability to neutralize them with antioxidants. This imbalance can lead to damage to sperm DNA, reduced sperm motility, and decreased sperm count, all of which can negatively impact fertility.

Antioxidants work by neutralizing free radicals, which are highly reactive molecules that can cause cellular damage. By reducing oxidative stress, antioxidants help to maintain the integrity of sperm DNA and improve overall sperm health. They also enhance sperm motility and increase sperm count, increasing the chances of successful fertilization.

Some of the most effective antioxidant supplements for improving male fertility include:

- **Vitamin C:** This powerful antioxidant helps to protect sperm from oxidative damage and improve sperm quality.

- **Vitamin E:** Another potent antioxidant that protects sperm cells from oxidative stress and improves sperm motility.
- **Selenium:** This mineral acts as an antioxidant and helps to maintain the structural integrity of sperm cells.
- **Zinc:** Essential for sperm production, zinc is an important antioxidant that plays a vital role in male fertility.
- **Coenzyme Q10:** This antioxidant helps to improve sperm motility and protect sperm cells from oxidative damage.

It's important to note that while antioxidant supplements can be beneficial for improving fertility, it's always best to consult with a healthcare professional before starting any new supplementation regimen. They can provide personalized recommendations based on your specific needs and ensure that you are taking the appropriate dosage.

Healthy Lifestyle Habits

When it comes to male fertility, adopting healthy lifestyle habits can have a significant impact on sperm quality and overall reproductive health. Diet, exercise, and stress reduction are three key areas to focus on when aiming to improve male fertility.

Diet: A balanced and nutritious diet plays a crucial role in enhancing fertility. Including foods rich in antioxidants, such as fruits, vegetables, and whole grains, can help protect sperm from oxidative damage. Additionally, consuming foods high in omega-3 fatty acids, such as fish, nuts, and seeds, may improve sperm motility and count. It is also important to limit the intake of processed foods, sugary beverages, and excessive caffeine, as they can negatively impact sperm health.

Exercise: Regular physical activity has been shown to improve male fertility. Engaging in moderate-intensity aerobic exercise, such as jogging or swimming, can help maintain a healthy weight and improve overall reproductive function. However, it is essential to avoid excessive exercise, as intense workouts may lead to increased scrotal temperatures, which can negatively affect sperm production.

Stress Reduction: Chronic stress can have a detrimental effect on male fertility. High levels of stress hormones, such as cortisol, can disrupt hormonal balance and reduce sperm production. Engaging in stress-reducing activities, such as meditation, yoga, or deep breathing exercises, can help lower stress levels and promote better reproductive health.

By adopting these healthy lifestyle habits, men can optimize their fertility potential and increase the chances of conception. It is important to remember that individual results may vary, and consulting with a healthcare professional is recommended for personalized advice and guidance.

Seeking Professional Help

When it comes to enhancing fertility, there may come a point where seeking professional help becomes necessary. Consulting a fertility specialist and exploring medical interventions can provide valuable insights and guidance on your journey towards conception. But how do you know when it's time to take this step?

There are several factors to consider when deciding to seek professional help. If you have been actively trying to conceive for a year or more without success, it may be a good idea to consult a fertility specialist. This timeframe is reduced to six months if you are over the age of 35, as fertility declines with age. Additionally, if you have a known medical condition that may affect fertility, such as polycystic ovary syndrome (PCOS) or endometriosis, it is advisable to seek professional guidance sooner rather than later.

A fertility specialist can offer a range of medical interventions to help improve your chances of conceiving. These may include fertility medications, such as Clomid or letrozole, which can stimulate ovulation. In some cases, assisted reproductive technologies like intrauterine insemination (IUI) or in vitro fertilization (IVF) may be recommended. These procedures involve the fertilization of eggs outside the body and their subsequent transfer into the uterus.

It is important to remember that seeking professional help does not mean giving up on natural remedies and holistic approaches. In fact, many fertility specialists integrate complementary therapies into their treatment plans to enhance their effectiveness. By combining the best of both worlds, you can optimize your chances of success and create a holistic approach to your fertility journey.

Natural Fertility Specialists

When it comes to fertility treatment, many individuals seek out the expertise of natural fertility specialists such as naturopathic doctors and holistic practitioners. These professionals take a holistic approach to fertility, focusing on the overall health and well-being of the individual rather than just treating the symptoms. They believe that by addressing the root causes of fertility issues and promoting overall health, they can enhance the chances of conception.

Naturopathic doctors are trained in both conventional medicine and natural therapies. They combine the best of both worlds to provide comprehensive care for their patients. These doctors take into account the individual's medical history, lifestyle factors, and emotional well-being to create a personalized treatment plan. They may recommend dietary changes, herbal supplements, acupuncture, and other natural therapies to support fertility.

Holistic practitioners, on the other hand, may include a variety of professionals such as acupuncturists, herbalists, nutritionists, and mind-body therapists. They work together to address the physical, emotional, and spiritual aspects of fertility. These practitioners often use alternative therapies, such as acupuncture and herbal medicine, to promote hormonal balance, improve reproductive health, and reduce stress.

One of the key advantages of working with natural fertility specialists is their emphasis on individualized care. They take the time to understand each person's unique situation and tailor their treatment approach accordingly. They recognize that fertility issues can stem from a variety of factors, including hormonal imbalances, nutritional deficiencies, stress, and environmental toxins. By addressing these factors, they aim to optimize fertility and increase the chances of conception.

In addition to providing personalized care, natural fertility specialists also prioritize education and empowerment. They strive to educate their patients about the underlying causes of their fertility issues and provide them with the tools and knowledge to make informed decisions about their health. They may offer guidance on lifestyle modifications, stress reduction techniques, and fertility-enhancing practices.

It is important to note that while natural fertility specialists can be valuable resources, they are not a substitute for medical advice. If you are experiencing fertility issues, it is essential to consult with a healthcare professional, such as a reproductive endocrinologist or a fertility specialist, to explore all available options. These specialists can provide a comprehensive evaluation, diagnose any underlying medical conditions, and recommend appropriate medical interventions if necessary.

In conclusion, natural fertility specialists, including naturopathic doctors and holistic practitioners, play a significant role in fertility treatment. They take a holistic approach to address the underlying causes of fertility issues and promote overall health and well-being. By providing individualized care, education, and empowerment, these specialists aim to enhance fertility and increase the chances of conception. However, it is important to work in conjunction with medical professionals to ensure a comprehensive approach to fertility treatment.

Assisted Reproductive Technologies

Assisted Reproductive Technologies (ART) offer a range of options for individuals and couples struggling with fertility issues. These advanced medical procedures can help overcome barriers to conception and increase the chances of achieving a successful pregnancy. Let's explore some of the different ART options available and their success rates.

1. In Vitro Fertilization (IVF): IVF is one of the most well-known and commonly used ART procedures. It involves the retrieval of eggs from the woman's ovaries and the fertilization of these eggs with sperm in a laboratory setting. The resulting embryos are then transferred back into the woman's uterus. IVF success rates vary depending on factors such as age, overall health, and the quality of the embryos. On average, the success rate for IVF is around 30-40% per cycle.

2. Intracytoplasmic Sperm Injection (ICSI): ICSI is a specialized form of IVF that is often recommended for couples dealing with male infertility issues. It involves the injection of a single sperm directly into an egg to facilitate fertilization. ICSI has shown high success rates, particularly in cases where male factor infertility is the primary concern.

3. Frozen Embryo Transfer (FET): FET involves the transfer of embryos that have been cryopreserved (frozen) from a previous IVF cycle. This procedure allows for the use of embryos at a later time, increasing the chances of a successful pregnancy. FET success rates can vary, but they are generally comparable to fresh embryo transfers.

4. Donor Egg or Sperm: For individuals or couples who are unable to produce viable eggs or sperm, donor eggs or sperm can be used in the ART process. Donor eggs are typically obtained from young, healthy women, while donor sperm is sourced from carefully screened donors. Success rates with donor eggs or sperm can be quite high, as they often come from individuals with excellent fertility potential.

5. Surrogacy: Surrogacy involves the use of a gestational carrier who carries and delivers a baby for individuals or couples who are unable to do so themselves. The intended parents may use their own eggs and sperm or opt for donor eggs or sperm. Success rates with surrogacy can vary depending on various factors, including the age and overall health of the surrogate.

It's important to note that success rates for ART procedures can be influenced by several factors, including the age of the woman, the quality of the eggs or sperm, the overall health of the individuals involved, and the experience and expertise of the fertility clinic. Consulting with a fertility specialist is crucial to understand which ART option is most suitable and to discuss the potential success rates based on individual circumstances.

Support and Community

Support and community play a crucial role in the fertility journey. Going through the ups and downs of trying to conceive can be emotionally challenging, and having a strong support system can provide the much-needed comfort and understanding. Connecting with others who are going through a similar experience can make you feel less alone and provide a sense of belonging.

One way to find support is by joining fertility support groups. These groups consist of individuals who are also on a fertility journey, and they provide a safe space to share experiences, emotions, and information. Being part of a support group allows you to connect with others who truly understand the rollercoaster of emotions that come with trying to conceive. You can gain valuable insights, learn coping strategies, and receive emotional support from people who have been through similar challenges.

In addition to support groups, online resources and forums can also be a valuable source of support. There are numerous online platforms where individuals can connect with others, share their experiences, and seek advice. These platforms provide a sense of community and allow you to connect with people from all over the world who are going through similar experiences. It can be comforting to know that you are not alone and that there are others who understand and can offer support.

Remember, seeking support and connecting with others on your fertility journey is not a sign of weakness, but rather a sign of strength. It takes courage to reach out and share your experiences with others. By building a support network, you can find solace, gain knowledge, and navigate the challenges of fertility with a sense of community.

Fertility Support Groups

Joining a fertility support group can provide valuable emotional and informational support for individuals and couples on their fertility journey. These groups offer a safe and understanding space where individuals can share their experiences, concerns, and emotions with others who are going through similar challenges.

One of the key benefits of joining a fertility support group is the opportunity to connect with others who truly understand the ups and downs of fertility struggles. It can be a relief to know that you are not alone in your experiences and that there are others who can empathize with your journey. Sharing your thoughts and feelings with others who are facing similar challenges can provide a sense of validation and comfort.

In addition to emotional support, fertility support groups also offer a wealth of information and resources. Members can share their knowledge about various fertility treatments, alternative therapies, and lifestyle changes that may improve fertility. This exchange of information can be invaluable in helping individuals make informed decisions about their own fertility journey.

Support groups can also provide a platform for individuals to learn from the experiences of others. Hearing success stories and learning about different coping strategies can inspire hope and provide motivation to continue on the path towards conception. It can also provide guidance on navigating the complex world of fertility treatments and medical interventions.

Furthermore, fertility support groups often invite guest speakers such as fertility specialists, nutritionists, and holistic practitioners to share their expertise. These professionals can provide valuable insights and answer questions that members may have about various aspects of fertility and reproductive health.

Whether it is in-person or online, joining a fertility support group can be a transformative experience. It offers a sense of belonging, understanding, and empowerment. By connecting with others who are on a similar journey, individuals and couples can find the strength and resilience to navigate the challenges of infertility.

Online Resources and Forums

Online Resources and Forums

When it comes to navigating the world of fertility, finding a supportive community can make all the difference. Online resources and forums provide a valuable platform for individuals to connect, share experiences, and find emotional support during their fertility journey.

One of the greatest advantages of online platforms is the ability to connect with others who are going through similar experiences. These communities offer a safe space where individuals can openly discuss their struggles, ask questions, and find comfort in knowing that they are not alone. Whether you are just starting your fertility journey or have been trying for some time, these online resources can provide a sense of camaraderie and understanding.

Additionally, online forums often feature expert advice and information from healthcare professionals, fertility specialists, and experienced individuals. These resources can be incredibly helpful in gaining knowledge about various fertility treatments, understanding the latest research, and learning about alternative therapies. From tips on natural remedies to discussions about assisted reproductive technologies, these forums offer a wealth of information that can empower individuals to make informed decisions.

Some online platforms also provide access to webinars, podcasts, and educational materials that delve deeper into fertility-related topics. These resources can be a valuable source of information for individuals who prefer to learn at their own pace and in the comfort of their own homes.

Whether you are seeking emotional support, educational resources, or a space to share your own experiences, online resources and forums can be a lifeline during your fertility journey. By connecting with others who understand your struggles and providing a wealth of information, these platforms can empower individuals to take control of their fertility and find hope for the future.

Frequently Asked Questions

- **What is acupuncture and how can it improve fertility?**

  Acupuncture is an ancient practice that involves inserting thin needles into specific points on the body. It can help regulate hormones, improve blood flow to the reproductive organs, reduce stress, and promote overall reproductive health. By addressing imbalances in the body, acupuncture can increase the chances of conception.

- **How do herbal supplements enhance fertility?**

  Herbal supplements, such as Vitex and Maca, have been used for centuries to support reproductive health. Vitex helps regulate menstrual cycles and promote ovulation, while Maca balances hormones and increases libido. These natural remedies can improve fertility by addressing hormonal imbalances and promoting optimal reproductive function.

- **Can exercise and yoga improve fertility?**

  Yes, physical activity and stress reduction techniques like yoga can have a positive impact on fertility. Fertility yoga incorporates specific poses that stimulate reproductive organs and promote hormonal balance. Regular cardiovascular exercise improves blood circulation, reduces stress, and enhances overall reproductive health.

- **What role does diet and nutrition play in enhancing fertility?**

A balanced diet and specific nutrients are crucial for fertility. Certain foods, such as leafy greens, berries, and nuts, contain fertility-enhancing properties. Adequate intake of vitamins, minerals, and antioxidants supports reproductive function. On the other hand, excessive consumption of sugar and processed foods can negatively affect fertility.

- **How can stress reduction techniques impact fertility?**

Stress can disrupt hormonal balance and affect fertility. Meditation is a powerful technique that calms the mind and balances hormones, promoting better fertility. Aromatherapy, using essential oils, can also reduce stress and promote reproductive health by creating a relaxing environment.

- **Are there alternative therapies that can enhance fertility?**

Yes, there are lesser-known therapies that can naturally enhance fertility. Mayan abdominal massage is an ancient technique that improves blood flow to the reproductive organs, supporting their optimal function. Castor oil packs can detoxify the body and improve fertility by reducing inflammation and promoting circulation.

- **What are endocrine disruptors and how do they affect fertility?**

Endocrine disruptors are chemicals found in everyday products that can disrupt hormonal balance and negatively impact fertility. These chemicals are commonly found in plastics, personal care products, and pesticides. Minimizing exposure to these toxins is important for maintaining reproductive health.

- **How can I enhance male fertility naturally?**

Male fertility can be improved through various natural remedies. Antioxidant supplements, such as vitamin C and zinc, protect sperm from oxidative damage and improve fertility. Adopting a healthy lifestyle, including a balanced diet, regular exercise, and stress reduction techniques, can also enhance male fertility.

- **When should I seek professional help for fertility issues?**

If you have been actively trying to conceive for a year without success (or six months if you're over 35), it may be time to consult a fertility specialist.

They can provide guidance, perform diagnostic tests, and explore medical interventions if necessary.

- **How can I find support and connect with others on a fertility journey?**

Joining a fertility support group can provide emotional and informational support during your fertility journey. These groups offer a safe space to share experiences, seek advice, and find encouragement. Additionally, online resources and forums dedicated to fertility provide a platform for connecting with others who are going through similar experiences.

Have Questions / Comments?

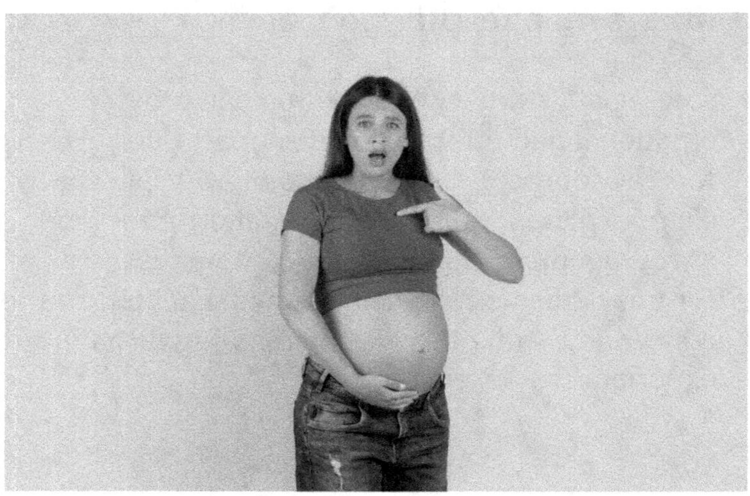

This book was designed to cover as much info as possible but I know I have probably missed something, or some new amazing discovery that has just come out.

If you notice something missing or have a question that I failed to answer, please get in touch and let me know. If I can, I will email you an answer and also update the book so others can also benefit from it.

Thanks For Being Awesome :)

Submit Your Questions / Comments At:

Get In Touch at Babydreamers.net

Get How To Be A Super Mom - 100% FREE

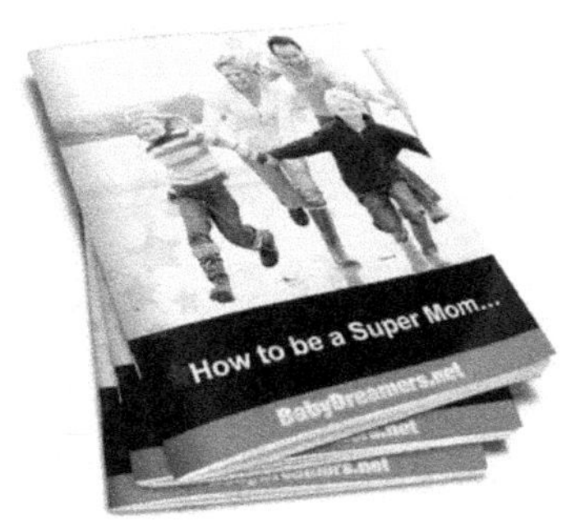

For being one of our amazing readers, we would love to offer you another book we have created, 100% free.

Being a mom is probably the most important job in the world – we've all heard that, and it's true. You're bringing up the next generation of wonderful, intelligent, loving, creative, responsible people.

We all want to be Super Mom and to be everything and do everything, but it this possible?

Being a Super Mom is possible, but you have to learn how to empower yourself to be the kind of Super Mom that you feel you need to be, keeping in mind that the title Super Mom doesn't mean the same thing to everyone.

Get How to be a Super Mom For Free at

BabyDreamers.net